METABOLIC CONFUSION DIET RECIPES

Complete Cookbook with Simple, Delicious Breakfast, Lunch, Dinner & Dessert Recipes to Boost Metabolism, Lose Weight, and Achieve Hormonal Balance.

Andrew H. Steve

About the Author

Andrew H. Steve, a renowned nutrition and health expert, specializes in empowering individuals to reclaim their health. With a passion for nutrition and a deep understanding of the human body and metabolism, Andrew has successfully guided many to achieve significant weight loss and enhanced well-being.

With over a decade of experience, Andrew's approach is far from one-size-fits-all. He tailors his advice to each individual, focusing on a holistic method that encompasses a balanced diet, mindful eating, and an active lifestyle, rather than just diets and restrictions.

Known for his ability to distill complex dietary concepts into practical, actionable strategies, Andrew is a guiding force in navigating the intricacies of metabolism and wellness. His dedication extends beyond his professional achievements, as he finds joy in outdoor activities, experimenting with new recipes, and engaging in healthy discussions.

If you're looking to lose weight, increase energy, or improve your overall well-being, Andrew H. Steve is your ideal mentor. Under his guidance, you're not just adopting a healthy lifestyle; you're embarking on a transformative journey to rediscover your vitality and thrive.

TABLE OF CONTENTS

CHAPTER 1

INTRODUCTION

Introduction to Metabolic Confusion

The concept of Metabolic Confusion is rooted in the idea of preventing the body from adapting to a consistent caloric intake, thus potentially enhancing metabolic efficiency and aiding in weight loss or management. This approach contrasts with traditional dieting methods, which often involve a consistent caloric deficit or specific macronutrient distribution.

Background and Principles

Traditional diets often lead to a plateau, a point where the body adapts to the reduced calorie intake and weight loss slows down or stops. Metabolic Confusion aims to circumvent this plateau by alternating between periods of higher and lower calorie consumption. This variation is believed to keep the metabolism active and prevent it from becoming efficient at operating on fewer calories.

How It Works

The Metabolic Confusion diet doesn't prescribe specific foods but focuses on calorie variation. Typically, it involves a cycle where a few days of lower calorie intake are followed by a few days of higher calorie intake. The 'low-calorie' days are designed to create a calorie deficit, promoting weight loss, while the 'high-calorie' days aim to boost metabolism and replenish energy.

Potential Benefits

1. **Avoiding Plateaus**: By constantly changing calorie intake, the body may not adapt as easily, potentially avoiding weight loss plateaus.

2. **Flexibility**: This diet offers more flexibility compared to strict calorie-controlled diets, making it easier for some people to adhere to in the long term.

3. **Psychological Benefits**: Higher calorie days can provide psychological relief from dieting, reducing the feeling of being constantly restricted.

Considerations and Criticisms

1. **Lack of Scientific Consensus**: There is limited scientific research specifically on Metabolic Confusion, so its effectiveness is still a subject of debate.

2. **Not a One-Size-Fits-All Solution**: Individual responses to calorie cycling can vary. For some, this approach may be less effective or harder to maintain.

3. **Importance of Nutritional Balance**: Regardless of calorie cycling, the importance of a balanced diet, including all macronutrients and essential vitamins and minerals, remains paramount.

Benefits and Principles of the Metabolic Confusion Diet

The Metabolic Confusion Diet, characterized by its alternating calorie intake approach, offers several potential benefits and is underpinned by certain principles. This approach contrasts with traditional constant-calorie diets, aiming to enhance metabolic efficiency and assist in weight management. Below, we'll explore the key benefits and principles of this diet.

Benefits of the Metabolic Confusion Diet

1. **Prevention of Metabolic Adaptation**: Traditional diets often result in a metabolic slowdown as the body adapts to consistent low-calorie intake. Metabolic Confusion seeks to prevent this by regularly changing calorie intake, potentially keeping the metabolism active.

2. **Avoiding Dietary Plateaus**: One of the most challenging aspects of weight loss is the plateau phase. By fluctuating calorie intake, the Metabolic Confusion

Diet aims to bypass these plateaus, potentially leading to sustained weight loss.

3. **Psychological Relief**: Strict diets can be mentally taxing. The higher calorie days in Metabolic Confusion provide a psychological break, making it easier for some people to stick with the diet long-term.

4. **Flexibility in Food Choices**: Unlike some diets that restrict certain foods, Metabolic Confusion focuses on calorie variation rather than specific foods or food groups, offering greater dietary flexibility.

5. **Improved Energy Levels**: Higher calorie days can help replenish energy stores, potentially leading to better overall energy levels, which is particularly beneficial for those engaging in regular physical activity.

Principles of the Metabolic Confusion Diet

1. **Calorie Cycling**: The core principle is alternating between higher and lower calorie days. This cycling is thought to prevent the body from adapting to a consistent calorie level.

2. **No Specific Food Restrictions**: The diet does not inherently restrict any food groups. The focus is on the

quantity (calories) rather than the type of food, though a balanced diet is still recommended for overall health.

3. **Adaptability to Individual Needs**: The diet can be tailored to individual preferences and lifestyles. The duration of low and high-calorie periods can vary based on personal goals and needs.

4. **Sustainability Over Short-Term Gains**: The approach promotes a potentially more sustainable way of dieting compared to extreme calorie restriction, which is difficult to maintain long-term.

5. **Balance and Nutritional Adequacy**: Despite the focus on calorie variation, it's important to maintain a balanced diet that provides essential nutrients, vitamins, and minerals.

CHAPTER 2

UNDERSTANDING METABOLIC CONFUSION

The Science Behind Metabolic Confusion

The concept of Metabolic Confusion, also known as calorie shifting or calorie cycling, is an eating pattern that alternates between periods of higher and lower caloric intake. This approach is based on the hypothesis that such variation can prevent the body from adapting to a consistent caloric intake, potentially boosting metabolism and aiding in weight management. Let's delve into the scientific basis behind this approach.

Understanding Metabolism and Adaptive Thermogenesis

To comprehend Metabolic Confusion, it's important to first understand basic metabolic processes and the concept of adaptive thermogenesis:

1. **Basal Metabolic Rate (BMR)**: This is the amount of energy expended while at rest. It accounts for the majority of daily caloric expenditure and is influenced by factors like age, sex, body size, and muscle mass.

2. **Adaptive Thermogenesis**: When caloric intake is significantly reduced (as in traditional diets), the body adapts by lowering its energy expenditure. This adaptive response, a form of metabolic slowdown, is a survival mechanism intended to conserve energy during times of caloric scarcity.

3. **Plateaus in Weight Loss**: This metabolic adaptation can lead to a plateau in weight loss, where further weight loss becomes difficult despite continued caloric restriction.

The Theory of Metabolic Confusion

The Metabolic Confusion diet aims to counteract the body's adaptive response:

1. **Preventing Metabolic Slowdown**: By alternating between lower and higher calorie days, the theory suggests that the body can be prevented from entering a state of metabolic efficiency (lower BMR), thus potentially avoiding or reducing the plateau effect in weight loss.

2. **Hormonal Responses**: Fluctuating caloric intake might influence hormones related to hunger and satiety, such

as ghrelin and leptin, potentially aiding in appetite control on low-calorie days.

Research and Evidence

The scientific evidence supporting Metabolic Confusion is mixed and still emerging. Some studies suggest that intermittent energy restriction (similar in concept to calorie cycling) can lead to weight loss and health improvements, comparable to continuous energy restriction. However, these studies often focus on fasting regimens, which are only somewhat analogous to Metabolic Confusion.

Criticisms and Limitations

1. **Lack of Direct Evidence**: There's a scarcity of direct, robust scientific studies specifically focusing on Metabolic Confusion. Much of the evidence is indirect, derived from studies on related dietary patterns like intermittent fasting.

2. **Individual Variability**: Metabolic responses to dieting can vary significantly among individuals, influenced by genetic, environmental, and lifestyle factors. What works for one person might not be as effective for another.

3. **Long-Term Sustainability and Health Impact**: The long-term effects and sustainability of Metabolic Confusion are not well-documented. Moreover, while calorie cycling focuses on quantity, the quality of the diet (nutrient density and variety) remains crucial for overall health.

Metabolic Confusion: Myth vs. Reality

The concept of Metabolic Confusion, also known as calorie shifting or calorie cycling, has garnered attention in the weight loss and fitness community. It's crucial to differentiate between what is supported by science (reality) and what remains speculative or exaggerated (myth). Let's explore both aspects to provide a clearer understanding of Metabolic Confusion.

Myth: Rapid and Effortless Weight Loss

Myth: Metabolic Confusion guarantees rapid and effortless weight loss. **Reality**: While calorie cycling may help prevent metabolic slowdown, it doesn't guarantee rapid weight loss. Effective weight loss typically requires a sustained caloric deficit, balanced nutrition, and often physical activity. The process varies considerably among individuals and is influenced by numerous factors like genetics, lifestyle, and overall diet quality.

Myth: Dramatic Metabolic Boost

Myth: This diet dramatically boosts metabolism, leading to higher calorie burning at rest. **Reality**: While the idea is to prevent a metabolic slowdown, there's no concrete evidence that Metabolic Confusion significantly boosts your basal metabolic rate (BMR). Metabolism is influenced by many factors, including age, muscle mass, and overall health, not just diet.

Reality: Prevention of Plateaus

Reality: One of the potential benefits of Metabolic Confusion is the avoidance of weight loss plateaus. By varying calorie intake, the body may not adapt as easily to a lower calorie level, which can happen in traditional, constant-calorie diets. However, this benefit varies among individuals.

Myth: One-Size-Fits-All Solution

Myth: Metabolic Confusion is suitable and effective for everyone. **Reality**: Responses to different dietary approaches vary widely among individuals. Some may find success with calorie cycling, while others may not notice significant benefits or might struggle with the inconsistency in daily calorie targets.

Reality: Psychological Ease and Flexibility

Reality: The diet can offer psychological relief and flexibility. Higher calorie days provide a break from the stricter low-calorie periods, which can make the diet easier to adhere to for some people. This flexibility can lead to a more sustainable approach to weight management in the long term.

Myth: No Need for Nutritional Balance

Myth: Since calorie cycling focuses on the number of calories, the quality of the diet isn't important. **Reality**: Regardless of calorie cycling, a balanced diet that provides essential nutrients, vitamins, and minerals is vital for overall health. The quality of calories consumed is as important as the quantity.

Reality: Limited Direct Scientific Evidence

Reality: There is a limited amount of direct, robust scientific research specifically focusing on Metabolic Confusion. While some studies suggest benefits of intermittent energy restriction, these are not directly equivalent to Metabolic Confusion and often focus on fasting regimens.

Planning Your Metabolic Confusion Diet

Planning a Metabolic Confusion Diet involves careful consideration to ensure it is balanced, sustainable, and tailored to individual needs. Here are 20 steps that can guide you through the process:

1. **Understand the Concept**: Familiarize yourself with the principles of Metabolic Confusion, including calorie cycling and its potential effects on metabolism.

2. **Assess Your Goals**: Define clear, realistic goals, whether it's weight loss, maintaining weight, or improving overall health.

3. **Consult a Healthcare Professional**: Before starting any new diet, especially if you have health concerns or conditions, consult a healthcare professional.

4. **Calculate Your Caloric Needs**: Determine your Basal Metabolic Rate (BMR) and Total Daily Energy Expenditure (TDEE) to understand your daily caloric needs.

5. **Establish Calorie Cycle Patterns**: Decide on the pattern of your calorie cycling, such as higher-calorie days interspersed with lower-calorie days. Common

patterns include 5:2 (five normal days, two low-calorie days) or alternating days.

6. **Plan Caloric Intake for Different Days**: Set specific calorie targets for high and low-calorie days based on your TDEE and goals.

7. **Ensure Nutritional Balance**: Plan meals that are balanced in macronutrients (proteins, fats, carbohydrates) and provide essential vitamins and minerals.

8. **Create a Meal Plan**: Develop a meal plan that fits your calorie targets for both high and low-calorie days. Include a variety of foods to keep it interesting and nutritionally balanced.

9. **Prepare Grocery Lists**: Make grocery lists that correspond with your meal plan to streamline your shopping and ensure you have all necessary ingredients.

10. **Learn Portion Sizes**: Understand and measure portion sizes to accurately meet your caloric goals.

11. **Schedule Your Meals and Snacks**: Plan your eating schedule – including meals and snacks – to evenly distribute your caloric intake throughout the day.

12. **Incorporate Hydration**: Ensure you are drinking enough water and staying hydrated.

13. **Track Your Food Intake**: Consider using a food diary or an app to track what you eat, especially to stay on track with your calorie cycling.

14. **Listen to Your Body**: Pay attention to your body's hunger and fullness cues. Adjust your plan if you consistently feel overly hungry or fatigued.

15. **Adjust as Needed**: Be prepared to adjust your calorie targets or cycling pattern based on your progress and how your body responds.

16. **Integrate Physical Activity**: Include regular physical activity into your routine, as it's an important part of overall health and weight management.

17. **Monitor Your Progress**: Regularly monitor your progress towards your goals, but focus on long-term trends rather than daily fluctuations.

18. **Stay Flexible**: Be willing to modify your plan as your lifestyle, goals, or health needs change.

19. **Seek Support if Needed**: Consider seeking support from nutritionists, dietitians, or support groups, especially if you find it challenging to stick to the plan.

20. **Evaluate Long-Term Sustainability**: Continuously assess the sustainability of the diet for your lifestyle. The goal is to find a balanced approach that can be maintained long-term.

Remember, the key to a successful Metabolic Confusion Diet, like any dietary plan, is ensuring it aligns with your individual health needs, lifestyle, and preferences. Adapting and fine-tuning your approach over time is essential for sustainability and effectiveness.

CHAPTER 3

THE RECIPES

Breakfast Recipes

Recipe 1: Low-Calorie Berry Smoothie

Ingredients: 1 cup mixed berries (frozen)

- ½ banana
- 1 cup spinach
- 1 cup almond milk (unsweetened)
- 1 tbsp chia seeds

Instructions:

1. Combine all ingredients in a blender.
2. Blend until smooth.

Nutritional Value: ~200 calories; 5g protein, 35g carbs, 4g fat

Serving Suggestions:

1. Top with a sprinkle of granola.
2. Serve with a side of herbal tea.

Recipe 2: High-Calorie Avocado Toast

Ingredients: 2 slices whole-grain bread

- 1 ripe avocado

- 2 eggs

- Salt and pepper to taste

- 1 tbsp olive oil

Instructions:

1. Toast the bread.

2. Mash the avocado and spread on toast.

3. Fry eggs in olive oil, season with salt and pepper, and place on top of avocado.

Nutritional Value: ~500 calories; 20g protein, 40g carbs, 30g fat

Serving Suggestions:

1. Add a side of fresh orange slices.

2. Serve with a glass of milk or a latte.

Recipe 3: Low-Calorie Greek Yogurt Parfait

Ingredients:

- 1 cup Greek yogurt (low-fat)

- ½ cup strawberries, sliced

- ¼ cup blueberries

- 1 tbsp honey

- 1 tbsp almond slivers

Instructions:

1. Layer Greek yogurt with berries in a glass.

2. Drizzle with honey and top with almond slivers.

Nutritional Value: ~250 calories; 15g protein, 35g carbs, 5g fat

Serving Suggestions:

1. Serve with a cup of green tea.

2. Accompany with a slice of whole-grain toast.

Recipe 4: High-Calorie Omelette

Ingredients:

- 3 eggs

- ¼ cup cheddar cheese, grated

- ¼ cup bell peppers, diced

- ¼ cup onions, diced

- 1 tbsp butter

Instructions:

1. Whisk eggs and pour into a buttered frying pan.

2. Add cheese, peppers, and onions; cook until set.

Nutritional Value: ~400 calories; 25g protein, 10g carbs, 30g fat

Serving Suggestions:

1. Serve with a side of roasted potatoes.

2. Accompany with a slice of whole-grain bread.

Recipe 5: Low-Calorie Oatmeal

Ingredients:

- ½ cup rolled oats

- 1 cup almond milk

- 1 apple, diced

- 1 tsp cinnamon

- 1 tbsp maple syrup

Instructions:

1. Cook oats in almond milk, add diced apple.

2. Stir in cinnamon and maple syrup.

Nutritional Value: ~250 calories; 6g protein, 50g carbs, 5g fat

Serving Suggestions:

1. Top with a dollop of low-fat Greek yogurt.

2. Serve with a cup of black coffee.

Recipe 6: High-Calorie Nutty Banana Pancakes

Ingredients:

- 1 cup whole wheat flour

- 1 ripe banana, mashed

- 1 egg

- 1 cup milk

- ¼ cup chopped walnuts

- 1 tsp baking powder

- 1 tbsp honey

- Butter for cooking

Instructions:

1. Mix flour, baking powder, mashed banana, egg, and milk to form a batter.

2. Stir in walnuts. Cook pancakes in a buttered skillet, flipping once.

3. Drizzle with honey before serving.

Nutritional Value: ~550 calories; 15g protein, 80g carbs, 20g fat

Serving Suggestions:

1. Serve with a dollop of Greek yogurt on top.

2. Pair with a glass of freshly squeezed orange juice.

Recipe 7: Low-Calorie Cottage Cheese and Pineapple Bowl

Ingredients:

- 1 cup low-fat cottage cheese

- 1/2 cup chopped pineapple

- 1 tbsp shredded coconut

- A sprinkle of cinnamon

Instructions:

1. Place cottage cheese in a bowl.

2. Top with pineapple, coconut, and a sprinkle of cinnamon.

Nutritional Value: ~200 calories; 25g protein, 20g carbs, 5g fat

Serving Suggestions:

1. Accompany with a slice of whole-grain toast.

2. Enjoy with a cup of herbal tea.

Recipe 8: High-Calorie Breakfast Burrito

Ingredients:

- 2 large whole wheat tortillas

- 4 eggs, scrambled

- ½ cup black beans, cooked

- ½ cup cheddar cheese, shredded

- ¼ cup salsa

- 1 avocado, sliced

- 1 tbsp olive oil

Instructions:

1. Cook scrambled eggs in olive oil.

2. Lay tortillas flat, top with eggs, black beans, cheese, salsa, and avocado.

3. Roll up and lightly grill on each side.

Nutritional Value: ~700 calories; 30g protein, 60g carbs, 40g fat

Serving Suggestions:

1. Serve with a side of sour cream or Greek yogurt.

2. Accompany with a fresh fruit salad.

Recipe 9: Low-Calorie Veggie Scramble

Ingredients:

- 2 eggs
- 1 cup spinach
- ½ cup cherry tomatoes, halved
- ¼ cup bell peppers, diced
- ¼ cup onions, diced
- 1 tsp olive oil
- Salt and pepper to taste

Instructions:

1. Sauté vegetables in olive oil until soft.

2. Add beaten eggs, scramble together until cooked.

3. Season with salt and pepper.

Nutritional Value: ~200 calories; 14g protein, 10g carbs, 12g fat

Serving Suggestions:

1. Serve with a slice of whole-grain toast.

2. Pair with a cup of green tea.

Recipe 10: High-Calorie Smoked Salmon Bagel

Ingredients:

- 1 whole grain bagel
- 3 oz smoked salmon
- 2 tbsp cream cheese
- ¼ red onion, thinly sliced
- 1 tbsp capers
- A few sprigs of fresh dill

Instructions:

1. Toast the bagel and spread with cream cheese.

2. Top with smoked salmon, onion slices, capers, and dill.

Nutritional Value: ~500 calories; 25g protein, 60g carbs, 20g fat

Serving Suggestions:

1. Serve with a side of cucumber and tomato salad.

2. Accompany with a glass of cold-pressed apple juice.

Recipe 11: Low-Calorie Chia Seed Pudding

Ingredients:

- 2 tbsp chia seeds
- 1 cup almond milk (unsweetened)
- ½ tsp vanilla extract
- 1 tbsp honey
- ½ cup mixed berries

Instructions:

1. Mix chia seeds with almond milk and vanilla extract. Let sit overnight in the fridge.

2. In the morning, stir the pudding, top with berries and drizzle with honey.

Nutritional Value: ~250 calories; 6g protein, 35g carbs, 10g fat

Serving Suggestions:

1. Pair with a small green smoothie.

2. Serve with a cup of herbal tea.

Recipe 12: High-Calorie Protein-Packed Breakfast Bowl

Ingredients:

- ½ cup cooked quinoa
- 2 eggs, boiled or poached
- ¼ avocado, sliced
- ½ cup spinach, steamed
- 1 tbsp olive oil
- Salt and pepper to taste

Instructions:

1. Arrange quinoa, eggs, avocado, and spinach in a bowl.
2. Drizzle with olive oil and season with salt and pepper.

Nutritional Value: ~600 calories; 25g protein, 45g carbs, 35g fat

Serving Suggestions:

1. Add a sprinkle of feta cheese.
2. Serve with a glass of fresh fruit juice.

Recipe 13: Low-Calorie Spinach and Mushroom Omelette

Ingredients: 2 eggs

- 1 cup spinach

- ½ cup mushrooms, sliced

- 1 tsp olive oil

- Salt and pepper to taste

Instructions:

1. Sauté mushrooms and spinach in olive oil.

2. Add beaten eggs and cook into an omelette. Season with salt and pepper.

Nutritional Value: ~200 calories; 14g protein, 6g carbs, 14g fat

Serving Suggestions:

1. Serve with a slice of whole-grain toast.

2. Pair with a cup of black coffee or tea.

Recipe 14: High-Calorie French Toast with Berries

Ingredients:

- 2 slices whole-grain bread

- 1 egg

- ½ cup milk

- ½ tsp cinnamon

- 1 tbsp butter

- ½ cup mixed berries

- 2 tbsp maple syrup

Instructions:

1. Whisk egg, milk, and cinnamon. Dip bread in the mixture.

2. Cook in buttered skillet on both sides until golden.

3. Top with berries and drizzle with maple syrup.

Nutritional Value: ~500 calories; 15g protein, 60g carbs, 20g fat

Serving Suggestions:

1. Serve with a dollop of Greek yogurt.

2. Accompany with a cup of cappuccino.

Recipe 15: Low-Calorie Turkey and Avocado Wrap

Ingredients:

- 1 whole-grain wrap
- 2 oz sliced turkey breast
- ¼ avocado, sliced
- ½ cup lettuce
- 1 tbsp Greek yogurt

Instructions:

1. Lay the wrap flat and spread Greek yogurt.

2. Add turkey, avocado slices, and lettuce. Roll up the wrap tightly.

Nutritional Value: ~250 calories; 20g protein, 25g carbs, 10g fat

Serving Suggestions:

1. Serve with a side of carrot and celery sticks.

2. Enjoy with a glass of tomato juice.

Recipe 16: High-Calorie Breakfast Hash

Ingredients:

- 1 medium potato, diced

- ½ cup bell peppers, diced

- ¼ cup onions, diced

- 2 eggs

- 2 sausage links, sliced

- 1 tbsp olive oil

- Salt and pepper to taste

Instructions:

1. Sauté potatoes, bell peppers, and onions in olive oil until tender.

2. Add sausage slices, cook until browned.

3. Make two wells, crack eggs into them, cover and cook until eggs are set.

Nutritional Value: ~700 calories; 25g protein, 50g carbs, 45g fat

Serving Suggestions:

1. Top with shredded cheese.

2. Serve with a slice of whole-grain toast.

Recipe 17: Low-Calorie Protein Shake

Ingredients:

- 1 scoop protein powder (any flavour)

- 1 cup almond milk (unsweetened)

- ½ banana

- 1 tbsp peanut butter

- Ice cubes

Instructions:

1. Blend all ingredients together until smooth.

Nutritional Value: ~250 calories; 25g protein, 20g carbs, 10g fat

Serving Suggestions:

1. Accompany with a small apple.

2. Enjoy with a handful of almonds.

Recipe 18: High-Calorie Eggs Benedict

Ingredients:

- 2 English muffins, halved and toasted

- 4 slices Canadian bacon

- 4 eggs, poached

- ½ cup hollandaise sauce

- 1 tbsp chopped parsley

Instructions:

1. Place bacon on muffin halves, top with poached eggs.

2. Drizzle with hollandaise sauce and garnish with parsley.

Nutritional Value: ~600 calories; 25g protein, 45g carbs, 40g fat

Serving Suggestions:

1. Serve with a side of roasted asparagus.

2. Pair with a mimosa or orange juice.

Recipe 19: Low-Calorie Cottage Cheese with Fresh Fruit

Ingredients:

- 1 cup low-fat cottage cheese

- ½ cup fresh pineapple, diced

- ½ cup fresh strawberries, sliced

- 1 tbsp honey

Instructions:

1. Mix cottage cheese with honey.

2. Top with diced pineapple and sliced strawberries.

Nutritional Value: ~200 calories; 20g protein, 25g carbs, 2g fat

Serving Suggestions:

1. Sprinkle with a dash of cinnamon.

2. Pair with a cup of green tea.

Recipe 20: High-Calorie Bagel with Lox

Ingredients:

- 1 whole-grain bagel

- 4 oz smoked salmon (lox)

- 2 tbsp cream cheese

- ¼ red onion, thinly sliced

- 1 tbsp capers

Instructions:

1. Toast the bagel and spread with cream cheese.

2. Add smoked salmon, onion, and capers on top.

Nutritional Value: ~500 calories; 30g protein, 50g carbs, 20g fat

Serving Suggestions:

1. Serve with a side of mixed greens.

2. Accompany with a glass of tomato juice or a bloody Mary.

Recipe 21: High-Calorie Huevos Rancheros

Ingredients: 2 corn tortillas

- 2 eggs
- ½ cup black beans, cooked
- ¼ cup salsa
- ¼ avocado, sliced
- 1 tbsp olive oil
- ¼ cup shredded cheese

Instructions:

1. Fry eggs in olive oil to your preference.
2. Warm tortillas, top with black beans, cooked eggs, salsa, avocado, and cheese.

Nutritional Value: ~600 calories; 25g protein, 50g carbs, 35g fat

Serving Suggestions:

1. Add a dollop of Greek yogurt on top.
2. Serve with a side of grilled tomato slices.

Recipe 22: Low-Calorie Almond Butter Toast

Ingredients: 2 slices whole-grain bread, toasted

- 2 tbsp almond butter

- ½ banana, sliced

- A sprinkle of chia seeds

Instructions:

1. Spread almond butter on toasted bread.

2. Top with banana slices and sprinkle with chia seeds.

Nutritional Value: ~300 calories; 10g protein, 40g carbs, 15g fat

Serving Suggestions:

1. Serve with a side of fresh berries.

2. Enjoy with a cup of black coffee.

Recipe 23: High-Calorie Breakfast Tacos

Ingredients:

- 2 small flour tortillas

- 3 eggs, scrambled

- ¼ cup chorizo, cooked

- ¼ cup cheddar cheese, shredded

- ¼ cup salsa

- 1 tbsp sour cream

Instructions:

1. Cook scrambled eggs and chorizo.

2. Fill tortillas with egg mixture, top with cheese, salsa, and sour cream.

Nutritional Value: ~700 calories; 30g protein, 40g carbs, 50g fat

Serving Suggestions:

1. Serve with a side of refried beans.

2. Pair with a glass of freshly squeezed orange juice.

Recipe 24: Low-Calorie Blueberry Yogurt Bowl

Ingredients:

- 1 cup Greek yogurt, low-fat

- ½ cup blueberries

- 1 tbsp honey

- A sprinkle of granola

Instructions:

1. Mix yogurt with honey.

2. Top with blueberries and a sprinkle of granola.

Nutritional Value: ~250 calories; 20g protein, 35g carbs, 5g fat

Serving Suggestions:

1. Serve with a side of cucumber slices.

2. Enjoy with a cup of herbal tea.

Recipe 25: High-Calorie Shakshuka

Ingredients: 4 eggs

- 1 can (14 oz) diced tomatoes

- ½ onion, diced

- 1 bell pepper, diced

- 2 garlic cloves, minced

- 2 tbsp olive oil

- 1 tsp paprika

- Salt and pepper to taste

- Fresh parsley for garnish

Instructions:

1. Sauté onion, bell pepper, and garlic in olive oil until soft.

2. Add tomatoes and paprika, simmer for 10 minutes.

3. Make wells in the sauce, crack eggs into them, cover, and cook until eggs are set.

4. Garnish with parsley.

Nutritional Value: ~500 calories; 20g protein, 40g carbs, 30g fat

Serving Suggestions:

1. Serve with a slice of whole-grain bread.

2. Pair with a cup of mint tea.

Recipe 26: Low-Calorie Apple Cinnamon Oats

Ingredients:

- ½ cup rolled oats

- 1 cup water or almond milk

- 1 apple, diced

- 1 tsp cinnamon

- 1 tbsp honey

Instructions:

1. Cook oats with water or almond milk.

2. Stir in diced apple and cinnamon.

3. Drizzle with honey before serving.

Nutritional Value: ~250 calories; 5g protein, 50g carbs, 5g fat

Serving Suggestions:

1. Top with a few walnuts or almonds.

2. Serve with a cup of green tea.

Recipe 27: High-Calorie Granola and Yogurt Parfait

Ingredients:

- 1 cup Greek yogurt, full-fat

- ½ cup granola

- 1/2 cup mixed berries

- 2 tbsp honey

Instructions:

1. Layer yogurt, granola, and berries in a glass.

2. Drizzle with honey.

Nutritional Value: ~500 calories; 20g protein, 60g carbs, 20g fat

Serving Suggestions:

1. Serve with a side of sliced banana.

2. Enjoy with a cup of chai latte.

Recipe 28: Low-Calorie Veggie and Egg White Scramble

Ingredients:

- 3 egg whites
- 1 cup spinach
- ½ cup cherry tomatoes, halved
- ¼ cup bell peppers, diced
- ¼ cup onions, diced
- 1 tsp olive oil
- Salt and pepper to taste

Instructions:

1. Sauté vegetables in olive oil until soft.

2. Add egg whites, scramble together until cooked.

3. Season with salt and pepper.

Nutritional Value: ~150 calories; 15g protein, 10g carbs, 5g fat

Serving Suggestions:

1. Serve with a slice of whole-grain toast.

2. Pair with a cup of black coffee.

Recipe 29: Low-Calorie Spinach and Feta Omelette

Ingredients:

- 3 egg whites

- 1 cup fresh spinach

- ¼ cup feta cheese, crumbled

- 1 tsp olive oil

- Salt and pepper to taste

Instructions:

1. Sauté spinach in olive oil until wilted.

2. Mix egg whites and pour over spinach. Sprinkle feta cheese.

3. Fold omelette and cook until egg whites are set.

Nutritional Value: ~200 calories; 18g protein, 5g carbs, 12g fat

Serving Suggestions:

1. Serve with a side of sliced tomatoes.

2. Pair with a cup of herbal tea.

Recipe 30: High-Calorie Peanut Butter and Banana Smoothie

Ingredients:

- 2 tbsp peanut butter

- 1 banana

- 1 cup whole milk

- 1 scoop protein powder (optional)

- Ice cubes

Instructions:

1. Blend all ingredients until smooth.

Nutritional Value: ~600 calories; 25g protein, 50g carbs, 30g fat

Serving Suggestions:

1. Accompany with a handful of trail mix.

2. Enjoy with a whole-grain bagel.

Recipe 31: Low-Calorie Tomato and Basil Bruschetta

Ingredients:

- 2 slices whole-grain bread, toasted

- 1 large tomato, diced

- 1 tbsp chopped fresh basil

- 1 tsp balsamic vinegar

- 1 garlic clove, minced

- Salt and pepper to taste

Instructions:

1. Combine tomato, basil, garlic, and balsamic vinegar.

2. Spoon mixture over toasted bread. Season with salt and pepper.

Nutritional Value: ~200 calories; 8g protein, 30g carbs, 5g fat

Serving Suggestions:

1. Serve with a side of cucumber slices.

2. Pair with a cup of green tea.

Recipe 32: High-Calorie Breakfast Smoothie Bowl

Ingredients:

- 1 frozen banana

- ½ cup mixed berries

- ½ cup Greek yogurt, full-fat

- ¼ cup granola

- 1 tbsp almond butter

- 1 tbsp honey

Instructions:

1. Blend banana, berries, and yogurt until smooth.

2. Pour into a bowl and top with granola, almond butter, and honey.

Nutritional Value: ~500 calories; 15g protein, 60g carbs, 25g fat

Serving Suggestions:

1. Sprinkle with chia seeds.

2. Serve with a side of sliced kiwi.

Recipe 33: Low-Calorie Avocado and Egg White Salad

Ingredients:

- 4 egg whites, boiled and chopped
- ½ avocado, diced
- ¼ cup cherry tomatoes, halved
- 1 tbsp lemon juice
- Salt and pepper to taste

Instructions:

1. Combine egg whites, avocado, and cherry tomatoes.

2. Drizzle with lemon juice, and season with salt and pepper.

Nutritional Value: ~250 calories; 20g protein, 15g carbs, 15g fat

Serving Suggestions:

1. Serve on a bed of mixed greens.

2. Pair with a cup of black coffee.

Recipe 34: High-Calorie Cream Cheese and Smoked Salmon Bagel

Ingredients:

- 1 whole-grain bagel

- 2 oz smoked salmon

- 2 tbsp cream cheese

- ¼ red onion, thinly sliced

- Capers (optional)

Instructions:

1. Toast the bagel and spread with cream cheese.

2. Top with smoked salmon, onion, and capers.

Nutritional Value: ~500 calories; 25g protein, 60g carbs, 20g fat

Serving Suggestions:

1. Serve with a side of fresh arugula salad.

2. Enjoy with a glass of cold-pressed apple juice.

Recipe 35: Low-Calorie Berry and Kiwi Fruit Salad

Ingredients:

- ½ cup strawberries, sliced

- ½ cup blueberries

- 1 kiwi, peeled and sliced

- 1 tbsp lemon juice

- 1 tsp honey

Instructions:

1. Combine all fruits in a bowl.

2. Drizzle with lemon juice and honey.

Nutritional Value: ~150 calories; 2g protein, 35g carbs, 1g fat

Serving Suggestions:

1. Top with a dollop of low-fat Greek yogurt.

2. Serve with a slice of whole-grain toast.

Recipe 36: High-Calorie Mediterranean Breakfast Pita

Ingredients:

- 1 whole wheat pita

- 2 eggs, scrambled

- ¼ cup feta cheese, crumbled

- ¼ cup spinach, sautéed

- ¼ cup roasted red peppers, chopped

- 1 tbsp olive oil

Instructions:

1. Scramble eggs in olive oil, adding spinach towards the end.

2. Stuff the pita with the egg mixture, feta cheese, and roasted red peppers.

Nutritional Value: ~550 calories; 20g protein, 45g carbs, 30g fat

Serving Suggestions:

1. Serve with a side of Greek yogurt.

2. Pair with a cup of black coffee.

These recipes are carefully crafted to provide a mix of flavours and nutritional profiles, suitable for different days of the Metabolic Confusion Diet. They emphasize variety and balance, ensuring a pleasing and sustainable dietary approach.

lunch Recipes

Recipe 1: Low-Calorie Tomato Basil Soup

Ingredients:

- 4 cups diced tomatoes
- 1 onion, chopped
- 2 cloves garlic, minced
- 2 cups vegetable broth
- ¼ cup fresh basil, chopped
- Salt and pepper to taste
- 1 tbsp olive oil

Instructions:

1. Sauté onion and garlic in olive oil until translucent.
2. Add tomatoes and broth, simmer for 20 minutes.
3. Blend until smooth, stir in basil, and season.

Nutritional Value: ~150 calories per serving

Serving Suggestions:

1. Accompany with a small garden salad.
2. Enjoy with a slice of whole-grain bread.

Recipe 2: High-Calorie Beef Stir-Fry

Ingredients:

- 200g thinly sliced beef

- 1 cup mixed bell peppers, sliced

- ½ cup broccoli florets

- 2 tbsp soy sauce

- 1 tbsp sesame oil

- 1 tsp ginger, grated

- 1 garlic clove, minced

- 1 cup cooked brown rice

Instructions:

1. Stir-fry beef, vegetables, ginger, and garlic in sesame oil.

2. Add soy sauce, cook until beef is done.

3. Serve over brown rice.

Nutritional Value: ~650 calories per serving

Serving Suggestions:

1. Pair with a cucumber salad.

2. Enjoy with a glass of iced green tea.

Recipe 3: Low-Calorie Cauliflower Rice Bowl

Ingredients:

- 2 cups cauliflower rice

- ½ cup black beans, cooked

- ½ avocado, sliced

- ¼ cup corn
- ¼ cup diced tomato
- Cilantro and lime for garnish
- Salt and pepper to taste

Instructions:

1. Cook cauliflower rice, season with salt and pepper.
2. Top with black beans, avocado, corn, and tomato.
3. Garnish with cilantro and lime.

Nutritional Value: ~300 calories per serving

Serving Suggestions:

1. Serve with a side of salsa.
2. Enjoy with a fruit-infused water.

Recipe 4: High-Calorie Chicken Caesar Wrap

Ingredients:

- 1 large whole wheat wrap
- 1 grilled chicken breast, sliced
- 1 cup romaine lettuce, chopped
- ¼ cup Caesar dressing
- 2 tbsp Parmesan cheese, grated
- ¼ cup croutons

Instructions:

1. Lay wrap flat, arrange chicken, lettuce, Parmesan, and croutons.

2. Drizzle with Caesar dressing, roll tightly.

Nutritional Value: ~600 calories per serving

Serving Suggestions:

1. Serve with a side of carrot sticks.

2. Pair with a cup of unsweetened iced tea.

Recipe 5: Low-Calorie Spinach and Goat Cheese Salad

Ingredients:

- 2 cups fresh spinach
- ¼ cup goat cheese, crumbled
- ¼ cup strawberries, sliced
- ¼ cup walnuts, chopped
- Balsamic vinaigrette dressing

Instructions:

1. Toss spinach with strawberries and walnuts.

2. Top with goat cheese and drizzle with dressing.

Nutritional Value: ~250 calories per serving

Serving Suggestions:

1. Accompany with a whole-grain roll.

2. Enjoy with a sparkling water.

Recipe 6: High-Calorie Tuna Pasta Salad

Ingredients:

- 2 cups cooked pasta
- 1 can tuna, drained
- ½ cup mayonnaise
- ¼ cup diced celery
- ¼ cup diced red onion
- Salt and pepper to taste
- 1 tbsp lemon juice

Instructions:

1. Mix tuna, mayonnaise, celery, onion, and lemon juice.
2. Combine with cooked pasta, season with salt and pepper.

Nutritional Value: ~700 calories per serving

Serving Suggestions:

1. Serve with a side of mixed greens.
2. Pair with a cup of herbal tea.

Recipe 7: Low-Calorie Greek Yogurt Chicken Salad

Ingredients:

- 1 grilled chicken breast, chopped
- ½ cup Greek yogurt
- ¼ cup grapes, halved
- ¼ cup almonds, sliced
- Salt and pepper to taste
- Lettuce leaves for serving

Instructions:

1. Combine chicken, yogurt, grapes, and almonds.
2. Season with salt and pepper.
3. Serve in lettuce leaves.

Nutritional Value: ~350 calories per serving

Serving Suggestions:

1. Enjoy with a side of cucumber slices.
2. Pair with a cup of green tea.

Recipe 8: High-Calorie Mediterranean Quinoa Bowl

Ingredients:

- 1 cup cooked quinoa
- ½ cup chickpeas, cooked
- ¼ cup feta cheese, crumbled
- ¼ cup Kalamata olives, sliced
- ½ cucumber, diced

- 1 tomato, diced

- Olive oil and lemon juice dressing

Instructions:

1. Combine quinoa with chickpeas, cucumber, tomato, and olives.

2. Mix in feta cheese and dress with olive oil and lemon juice.

Nutritional Value: ~600 calories per serving

Serving Suggestions:

1. Serve with a side of pita bread.

2. Enjoy with a glass of iced mint tea.

Recipe 9: Low-Calorie Veggie Wrap

Ingredients:

- 1 whole wheat wrap

- ½ cup hummus

- ¼ cup bell pepper, sliced

- ¼ cup carrot, julienned

- ¼ cup cucumber, sliced

- ¼ cup mixed greens

Instructions:

1. Spread hummus on the wrap.

2. Add vegetables and greens, roll tightly.

Nutritional Value: ~300 calories per serving

Serving Suggestions:

1. Serve with a side of fruit salad.

2. Pair with a cup of flavoured sparkling water.

Recipe 10: High-Calorie Turkey and Cheese Panini

Ingredients:

- 2 slices sourdough bread
- 4 slices turkey breast
- 2 slices Swiss cheese
- 1 tbsp mustard
- 1 tbsp mayonnaise
- ¼ avocado, sliced

Instructions:

1. Assemble sandwich with turkey, cheese, avocado, mustard, and mayonnaise.

2. Grill in a panini press until golden.

Nutritional Value: ~650 calories per serving

Serving Suggestions:

1. Serve with a side of baked potato wedges.

2. Enjoy with a cup of lemonade.

Recipe 11: Low-Calorie Zucchini Noodles with Tomato Sauce

Ingredients:

- 2 medium zucchinis, spiralized
- 1 cup tomato sauce
- 1 garlic clove, minced
- 1 tbsp olive oil
- Salt and pepper to taste
- Fresh basil for garnish

Instructions:

1. Sauté garlic in olive oil, add tomato sauce, simmer for 10 minutes.
2. Toss zucchini noodles in the sauce for 2-3 minutes.
3. Season with salt, pepper, and garnish with basil.

Nutritional Value: ~200 calories per serving

Serving Suggestions:

1. Top with a sprinkle of nutritional yeast.
2. Enjoy with a side salad.

Recipe 12: High-Calorie Chicken and Avocado Club Sandwich

Ingredients:

- 3 slices of whole-grain bread, toasted

- 2 grilled chicken breasts, sliced

- 1 avocado, mashed

- 2 lettuce leaves

- 2 tomato slices

- 2 bacon strips, cooked

- 1 tbsp mayonnaise

Instructions:

1. Layer one slice of bread with chicken, lettuce, tomato, and bacon.

2. Add second slice of bread, spread with avocado, top with remaining ingredients and bread.

Nutritional Value: ~800 calories per serving

Serving Suggestions:

1. Serve with a handful of baked potato chips.

2. Pair with a fruit smoothie.

Recipe 13: Low-Calorie Broccoli and Carrot Slaw

Ingredients:

- 2 cups broccoli, shredded

- 1 carrot, shredded

- ¼ red onion, thinly sliced

- 2 tbsp Greek yogurt

- 1 tbsp apple cider vinegar

- Salt and pepper to taste

Instructions:

1. Mix broccoli, carrot, and onion.

2. Dress with Greek yogurt and vinegar, season.

Nutritional Value: ~150 calories per serving

Serving Suggestions:

1. Accompany with a slice of whole-grain toast.

2. Enjoy with a cup of herbal tea.

Recipe 14: High-Calorie Shrimp and Mango Salad

Ingredients:

- 1 cup cooked shrimp

- 1 mango, diced

- ½ cucumber, diced

- ¼ red bell pepper, diced

- ¼ cup cilantro, chopped

- Lime juice and olive oil dressing

- Salt and pepper to taste

Instructions:

1. Combine shrimp, mango, cucumber, bell pepper, and cilantro.

2. Dress with lime juice and olive oil, season.

Nutritional Value: ~600 calories per serving

Serving Suggestions:

1. Serve over a bed of arugula.

2. Pair with a glass of iced tea.

Recipe 15: Low-Calorie Egg and Spinach Frittata

Ingredients:

- 4 egg whites

- 1 cup spinach, chopped

- ¼ cup mushrooms, sliced

- ¼ cup red bell pepper, diced

- 1 garlic clove, minced

- Salt and pepper to taste

- 1 tsp olive oil

Instructions:

1. Sauté garlic, bell pepper, mushrooms, and spinach in oil.

2. Pour egg whites over vegetables, cook until set.

Nutritional Value: ~200 calories per serving

Serving Suggestions:

1. Enjoy with a tomato cucumber salad.

2. Pair with a cup of green tea.

Recipe 16: High-Calorie Beef and Cheese Quesadilla

Ingredients:

- 2 large whole wheat tortillas
- ½ cup cooked ground beef
- ½ cup cheddar cheese, shredded
- ¼ cup black beans
- ¼ cup corn
- Salsa and sour cream for serving

Instructions:

1. Spread beef, cheese, beans, and corn between tortillas.
2. Cook in a skillet until cheese melts and tortilla is crispy.
3. Serve with salsa and sour cream.

Nutritional Value: ~700 calories per serving

Serving Suggestions:

1. Serve with a side of guacamole.
2. Enjoy with a glass of lemonade.

Recipe 17: Low-Calorie Cauliflower Steak

Ingredients:

- 1 large cauliflower, sliced into steaks

- 1 tbsp olive oil

- 1 tsp smoked paprika

- Salt and pepper to taste

- Lemon wedges for serving

Instructions:

1. Brush cauliflower steaks with olive oil and season.

2. Grill or bake until tender.

3. Serve with lemon wedges.

Nutritional Value: ~150 calories per serving

Serving Suggestions:

1. Accompany with a quinoa salad.

2. Pair with a glass of sparkling water.

Recipe 18: High-Calorie Pork Chop with Apple Chutney

Ingredients:

- 1 large pork chop

- 1 apple, diced

- ¼ onion, diced

- 1 tbsp cider vinegar

- 1 tbsp brown sugar

- 1 tsp olive oil

- Salt and pepper to taste

Instructions:

1. Season pork chop, pan-sear in oil until cooked.

2. Sauté apple and onion, add vinegar and sugar, simmer into chutney.

3. Serve pork chop topped with chutney.

Nutritional Value: ~650 calories per serving

Serving Suggestions:

1. Serve with a side of roasted sweet potatoes.

2. Enjoy with a glass of apple cider.

Recipe 19: Low-Calorie Vegan Buddha Bowl

Ingredients:

- ½ cup chickpeas, cooked

- ½ cup quinoa, cooked

- ½ cup roasted vegetables (carrots, Brussels sprouts)

- ¼ avocado, sliced

- Tahini dressing

- Salt and pepper to taste

Instructions:

1. Arrange chickpeas, quinoa, vegetables, and avocado in a bowl.

2. Drizzle with tahini dressing, season.

Nutritional Value: ~400 calories per serving

Serving Suggestions:

1. Top with a sprinkle of sesame seeds.

2. Pair with a cup of kombucha.

Recipe 20: High-Calorie Italian Meatball Sub

Ingredients:

- 4 cooked meatballs in marinara sauce

- 1 sub roll

- ¼ cup mozzarella cheese, shredded

- 1 tbsp Parmesan cheese, grated

- Fresh basil leaves

Instructions:

1. Place meatballs and sauce in sub roll.

2. Top with mozzarella and Parmesan.

3. Broil until cheese is melted and bubbly.

4. Garnish with basil leaves.

Nutritional Value: ~800 calories per serving

Serving Suggestions:

1. Serve with a side of Caesar salad.

2. Enjoy with a glass of iced tea.

Recipe 21: Low-Calorie Mediterranean Chickpea Salad

Ingredients: 1 cup chickpeas, drained and rinsed

- ½ cucumber, diced
- ½ red bell pepper, diced
- ¼ red onion, thinly sliced
- 2 tbsp feta cheese, crumbled
- 1 tbsp olive oil
- Lemon juice, salt, and pepper to taste

Instructions:

1. Combine chickpeas, cucumber, bell pepper, and onion in a bowl.
2. Drizzle with olive oil and lemon juice, season with salt and pepper.
3. Sprinkle with feta cheese before serving.

Nutritional Value: ~350 calories per serving

Serving Suggestions:

1. Serve over a bed of fresh spinach.
2. Pair with a glass of sparkling water with a lemon wedge.

Recipe 22: High-Calorie BBQ Chicken Pizza

Ingredients: 1 pre-made pizza base

- ½ cup BBQ sauce

- 1 grilled chicken breast, shredded

- ½ red onion, thinly sliced

- 1 cup mozzarella cheese, shredded

- Fresh cilantro for garnish

Instructions:

1. Spread BBQ sauce on the pizza base.

2. Top with chicken, red onion, and mozzarella cheese.

3. Bake according to pizza base instructions.

4. Garnish with fresh cilantro after baking.

Nutritional Value: ~800 calories per serving

Serving Suggestions:

1. Serve with a side of mixed greens salad.

2. Enjoy with a cold iced tea.

Recipe 23: Low-Calorie Asian Cabbage Salad

Ingredients:

- 2 cups shredded cabbage

- 1 carrot, julienned

- ½ bell pepper, thinly sliced

- ¼ cup edamame

- 1 tbsp sesame seeds

- 2 tbsp soy sauce

- 1 tbsp rice vinegar

- 1 tsp honey

- 1 tsp sesame oil

Instructions:

1. Mix cabbage, carrot, bell pepper, and edamame in a bowl.

2. Whisk together soy sauce, vinegar, honey, and sesame oil for the dressing.

3. Toss the salad with the dressing and sprinkle with sesame seeds.

Nutritional Value: ~200 calories per serving

Serving Suggestions:

1. Pair with a small portion of grilled chicken.

2. Enjoy with a cup of green tea.

Recipe 24: High-Calorie Creamy Pasta with Bacon

Ingredients:

- 2 cups cooked pasta

- 4 strips of bacon, cooked and chopped

- ½ cup heavy cream

- ¼ cup Parmesan cheese, grated

- 1 garlic clove, minced

- Salt and pepper to taste

- Fresh parsley, chopped for garnish

Instructions:

1. In a pan, cook garlic, add cream, and simmer.

2. Stir in Parmesan cheese until melted.

3. Add cooked pasta and bacon, season with salt and pepper.

4. Garnish with parsley before serving.

Nutritional Value: ~750 calories per serving

Serving Suggestions:

1. Serve with a side of garlic bread.

2. Pair with a glass of red wine.

Recipe 25: Low-Calorie Stuffed Bell Peppers

Ingredients:

- 2 bell peppers, halved and seeded

- ½ cup quinoa, cooked

- ¼ cup black beans, cooked

- ¼ cup corn

- ½ cup tomato sauce

- 1 tsp cumin

- Salt and pepper to taste

Instructions:

1. Mix quinoa, black beans, corn, tomato sauce, and cumin.

2. Stuff the bell peppers with the mixture.

3. Bake at 375°F for 25-30 minutes.

Nutritional Value: ~300 calories per serving

Serving Suggestions:

1. Top with a dollop of Greek yogurt.

2. Serve with a side of salsa.

Recipe 26: High-Calorie Steak and Potato Salad

Ingredients:

- 1 grilled steak, sliced

- 2 cups mixed salad greens

- ½ cup cherry tomatoes, halved

- 1 cup roasted potatoes, cubed

- ¼ cup blue cheese, crumbled

- Balsamic vinaigrette dressing

Instructions:

1. Arrange salad greens on a plate.

2. Top with steak, tomatoes, potatoes, and blue cheese.

3. Drizzle with balsamic vinaigrette.

Nutritional Value: ~650 calories per serving

Serving Suggestions:

1. Serve with a Side of Roasted Vegetables

2. Pair with a Glass of Red Wine

Recipe 27: Low-Calorie Turkey Lettuce Wraps

Ingredients: 200g ground turkey

- 1 bell pepper, diced

- 1 onion, diced

- 1 garlic clove, minced

- 1 tsp soy sauce

- 1 head iceberg lettuce

- 1 tbsp olive oil

- Salt and pepper to taste

Instructions:

1. Sauté onion and garlic in olive oil. Add turkey and cook until browned.

2. Stir in bell pepper and soy sauce, cook for a few minutes.

3. Spoon the mixture into lettuce leaves and wrap.

Nutritional Value: ~300 calories per serving

Serving Suggestions:

1. Pair with a side of cucumber slices.

2. Enjoy with a cup of herbal tea.

Recipe 28: High-Calorie Chicken Alfredo Pasta

Ingredients: 2 cups cooked fettuccine pasta

- 1 grilled chicken breast, sliced
- ½ cup Alfredo sauce
- ¼ cup Parmesan cheese
- 1 tbsp butter
- Salt and pepper to taste
- Fresh parsley for garnish

Instructions:

1. Heat Alfredo sauce in a pan, add butter and Parmesan cheese.
2. Toss cooked pasta and sliced chicken in the sauce.
3. Season with salt and pepper, and garnish with parsley.

Nutritional Value: ~700 calories per serving

Serving Suggestions:

1. Serve with a side of garlic bread.
2. Pair with a glass of white wine.

Recipe 29: Low-Calorie Veggie Sushi Rolls

Ingredients: 1 cup cooked sushi rice, cooled

- 2 nori sheets

- ¼ cucumber, julienned

- ¼ avocado, sliced

- ¼ red bell pepper, julienned

- Soy sauce for dipping

Instructions:

1. Spread rice evenly over nori sheets.

2. Place cucumber, avocado, and bell pepper on top.

3. Roll tightly and slice into sushi pieces.

Nutritional Value: ~250 calories per serving

Serving Suggestions:

1. Serve with soy sauce for dipping.

2. Pair with a side of pickled ginger and wasabi.

Recipe 30: High-Calorie Pulled Pork Sandwich

Ingredients:

- 200g pulled pork

- 1 large bun, halved

- ¼ cup BBQ sauce

- 1/4 cup coleslaw

- 1 tbsp mayonnaise

Instructions:

1. Mix pulled pork with BBQ sauce.

2. Spread mayonnaise on the bun, add pork, and top with coleslaw.

Nutritional Value: ~800 calories per serving

Serving Suggestions:

1. Serve with a side of baked beans.

2. Enjoy with a glass of root beer.

Recipe 31: Low-Calorie Grilled Veggie and Hummus Sandwich

Ingredients: 2 slices whole-grain bread, ¼ cup hummus

- ½ zucchini, sliced and grilled

- ½ red bell pepper, grilled

- ¼ red onion, grilled , 1 handful baby spinach

Instructions:

1. Spread hummus on bread slices.

2. Layer grilled vegetables and spinach between the bread.

Nutritional Value: ~350 calories per serving

Serving Suggestions:

1. Pair with a side of carrot and celery sticks.

2. Enjoy with a cup of iced green tea.

Recipe 1: Low-Calorie Grilled Salmon with Asparagus

Ingredients:

- 1 salmon fillet
- 1 bunch asparagus
- 1 lemon, sliced
- Salt, pepper, and dill to taste
- 1 tsp olive oil

Instructions:

1. Season salmon with salt, pepper, and dill.
2. Grill salmon and asparagus, drizzling asparagus with olive oil.
3. Serve with lemon slices.

Nutritional Value: ~300 calories per serving

Serving Suggestions:

1. Pair with a mixed greens salad.
2. Enjoy with a glass of sparkling water with a lemon wedge.

Recipe 2: High-Calorie Beef and Vegetable Stir-Fry

Ingredients:

- 200g beef strips

- 1 cup mixed vegetables (broccoli, bell peppers, carrots)

- 2 tbsp soy sauce

- 1 tbsp sesame oil

- 1 tsp ginger, grated

- 1 garlic clove, minced

- 1 cup cooked brown rice

Instructions:

1. Stir-fry beef and vegetables in sesame oil with ginger and garlic.

2. Add soy sauce, cook until beef is done.

3. Serve over brown rice.

Nutritional Value: ~700 calories per serving

Serving Suggestions:

1. Serve with a side of kimchi.

2. Enjoy with a cold beer or iced green tea.

Recipe 3: Low-Calorie Baked Cod with Lemon and Herbs

Ingredients:

- 2 cod fillets

- 1 lemon, sliced

- 1 tbsp olive oil

- Mixed herbs (thyme, parsley)
- Salt and pepper to taste

Instructions:

1. Place cod on a baking sheet, season with herbs, salt, and pepper.
2. Drizzle with olive oil and top with lemon slices.
3. Bake at 375°F for 20 minutes.

Nutritional Value: ~250 calories per serving

Serving Suggestions:

1. Accompany with a quinoa salad.
2. Pair with a glass of white wine.

Recipe 4: High-Calorie Creamy Chicken Alfredo

Ingredients:

- 2 chicken breasts, grilled and sliced
- 2 cups cooked fettuccine pasta
- ½ cup Alfredo sauce
- ¼ cup Parmesan cheese
- 1 tbsp butter
- Salt and pepper to taste
- Fresh parsley for garnish

Instructions:

1. Heat Alfredo sauce in a pan, add butter and Parmesan cheese.

2. Toss cooked pasta and sliced chicken in the sauce.

3. Season with salt and pepper, and garnish with parsley.

Nutritional Value: ~800 calories per serving

Serving Suggestions:

1. Serve with a side of garlic bread.

2. Pair with a glass of Chardonnay.

Recipe 5: Low-Calorie Vegetable Curry

Ingredients:

- 1 cup cauliflower florets

- ½ cup chickpeas, cooked

- ½ cup diced tomatoes

- ½ cup coconut milk

- 1 tbsp curry powder

- Salt to taste

- 1 tsp olive oil

Instructions:

1. Sauté cauliflower and chickpeas in olive oil.

2. Add tomatoes, coconut milk, and curry powder, simmer until vegetables are tender.

3. Season with salt.

Nutritional Value: ~350 calories per serving

Serving Suggestions:

1. Serve over a small portion of brown rice.

2. Enjoy with a side of cucumber raita.

Recipe 6: High-Calorie Pork Chop with Apple Sauce

Ingredients:

- 2 pork chops

- 2 apples, peeled and diced

- ¼ onion, diced

- 1 tbsp brown sugar

- 1 tsp cinnamon

- Salt and pepper to taste

- 1 tbsp olive oil

Instructions:

1. Season pork chops with salt and pepper, sear in olive oil until cooked.

2. In the same pan, cook apples, onion, sugar, and cinnamon until a sauce forms.

3. Serve pork chops topped with apple sauce.

Nutritional Value: ~650 calories per serving

Serving Suggestions:

1. Pair with roasted sweet potatoes.

2. Serve with a glass of red wine or apple cider.

Recipe 7: Low-Calorie Stuffed Bell Peppers

Ingredients:

- 4 bell peppers, halved and seeded
- 1 cup cooked quinoa
- ½ cup black beans
- ½ cup corn
- ½ cup tomato sauce
- 1 tsp cumin
- Salt and pepper to taste

Instructions:

1. Mix quinoa, black beans, corn, and tomato sauce, season with cumin, salt, and pepper.

2. Stuff bell peppers with the mixture.

3. Bake at 375°F for 25 minutes.

Nutritional Value: ~300 calories per serving

Serving Suggestions:

1. Serve with a side of salsa or Greek yogurt.

2. Enjoy with a glass of iced herbal tea.

Recipe 8: High-Calorie Lasagna

Ingredients:

- Lasagna noodles, cooked
- ½ lb ground beef
- 1 cup marinara sauce
- 1 cup ricotta cheese
- 1 cup mozzarella cheese, shredded
- ¼ cup Parmesan cheese, grated
- 1 egg
- Salt, pepper, and Italian seasoning

Instructions:

1. Brown ground beef, mix with marinara sauce.
2. Combine ricotta, egg, salt, and pepper.
3. Layer noodles, meat sauce, ricotta mixture, and mozzarella in a baking dish.
4. Top with Parmesan and bake at 375°F for 45 minutes.

Nutritional Value: ~800 calories per serving

Serving Suggestions:

1. Serve with a Caesar salad.

2. Enjoy with a glass of Sangiovese wine.

Recipe 9: Low-Calorie Lemon Garlic Shrimp

Ingredients: 200g shrimp, peeled and deveined

- 2 garlic cloves, minced
- 1 lemon, juice and zest
- Salt and pepper to taste
- 1 tbsp olive oil
- Fresh parsley, chopped

Instructions:

1. Marinate shrimp in lemon juice, zest, garlic, salt, and pepper.
2. Sauté shrimp in olive oil until cooked.
3. Garnish with parsley.

Nutritional Value: ~250 calories per serving

Serving Suggestions:

1. Serve over a bed of zucchini noodles.
2. Pair with a glass of Sauvignon Blanc.

Recipe 10: High-Calorie Beef Stroganoff

Ingredients:

- 300g beef strips
- 1 onion, chopped

- 1 cup mushrooms, sliced

- 1 cup sour cream

- 2 tbsp flour

- 2 cups beef broth

- Salt and pepper to taste

- 1 tbsp olive oil

- Cooked egg noodles

Instructions:

1. Brown beef in olive oil, set aside.

2. Sauté onion and mushrooms, stir in flour.

3. Add broth, bring to a simmer. Return beef to the pan.

4. Stir in sour cream, season with salt and pepper.

5. Serve over egg noodles.

Nutritional Value: ~750 calories per serving

Serving Suggestions:

1. Pair with a side of steamed green beans.

2. Enjoy with a dark beer or a glass of red wine.

Recipe 11: Low-Calorie Grilled Eggplant and Zucchini

Ingredients:

- 1 eggplant, sliced

- 2 zucchinis, sliced

- 2 tbsp olive oil

- 1 tsp garlic powder

- Salt and pepper to taste

- Fresh herbs (basil or parsley) for garnish

Instructions:

1. Brush eggplant and zucchini slices with olive oil, sprinkle with garlic powder, salt, and pepper.

2. Grill until tender.

3. Garnish with fresh herbs.

Nutritional Value: ~200 calories per serving

Serving Suggestions:

1. Pair with a quinoa salad.

2. Enjoy with a glass of lemon-infused water.

Recipe 12: High-Calorie Shrimp Alfredo Pasta

Ingredients:

- 200g cooked shrimp

- 2 cups cooked fettuccine

- ½ cup Alfredo sauce

- ¼ cup Parmesan cheese

- 1 tbsp butter

- Salt and pepper to taste

- Fresh parsley for garnish

Instructions:

1. Heat Alfredo sauce in a pan, add butter and Parmesan cheese.

2. Toss in cooked shrimp and pasta, season with salt and pepper.

3. Garnish with parsley before serving.

Nutritional Value: ~700 calories per serving

Serving Suggestions:

1. Serve with a side of steamed broccoli.

2. Pair with a glass of Chardonnay.

Recipe 13: Low-Calorie Baked Lemon Chicken

Ingredients:

- 2 chicken breasts

- 1 lemon, juiced and zested

- 2 garlic cloves, minced

- 1 tsp dried thyme

- Salt and pepper to taste

- 1 tbsp olive oil

Instructions:

1. Marinate chicken in lemon juice, zest, garlic, thyme, salt, and pepper.

2. Bake in preheated oven at 375°F for 25-30 minutes.

3. Drizzle with olive oil before serving.

Nutritional Value: ~250 calories per serving

Serving Suggestions:

1. Accompany with a mixed greens salad.

2. Enjoy with a cup of herbal tea.

Recipe 14: High-Calorie Beef Chili

Ingredients:

- 500g ground beef
- 1 can kidney beans, drained
- 1 can diced tomatoes
- 1 onion, chopped
- 2 garlic cloves, minced
- 1 tbsp chili powder
- Salt and pepper to taste
- 1 tbsp olive oil

Instructions:

1. Brown beef with onion and garlic in olive oil.

2. Add beans, tomatoes, chili powder, season with salt and pepper.

3. Simmer for 30 minutes.

Nutritional Value: ~800 calories per serving

Serving Suggestions:

1. Top with shredded cheddar cheese and sour cream.

2. Serve with a side of cornbread.

Recipe 15: Low-Calorie Tofu and Broccoli Stir-Fry

Ingredients:

- 1 block firm tofu, cubed

- 2 cups broccoli florets

- 2 tbsp soy sauce

- 1 tsp ginger, grated

- 1 garlic clove, minced

- 1 tsp sesame oil

- Sesame seeds for garnish

Instructions:

1. Stir-fry tofu in sesame oil until golden.

2. Add broccoli, garlic, ginger, and soy sauce, cook until broccoli is tender.

3. Garnish with sesame seeds.

Nutritional Value: ~350 calories per serving

Serving Suggestions:

1. Serve over a small portion of brown rice.

2. Enjoy with a cup of green tea.

Recipe 16: High-Calorie Lamb Curry

Ingredients:

- 500g lamb, cubed
- 1 onion, chopped
- 2 garlic cloves, minced
- 1 tbsp curry powder
- 1 can coconut milk
- 1 cup diced tomatoes
- Salt to taste
- 1 tbsp vegetable oil

Instructions:

1. Brown lamb with onion and garlic in oil.
2. Add curry powder, coconut milk, and tomatoes, simmer until lamb is tender.
3. Season with salt.

Nutritional Value: ~750 calories per serving

Serving Suggestions:

1. Serve with a side of basmati rice.
2. Pair with a cucumber raita.

Recipe 17: Low-Calorie Mushroom and Spinach Frittata

Ingredients:

- 4 egg whites
- 1 cup mushrooms, sliced
- 1 cup spinach, chopped
- ¼ cup onions, diced
- Salt and pepper to taste
- 1 tsp olive oil

Instructions:

1. Sauté mushrooms, spinach, and onions in olive oil.
2. Pour egg whites over the vegetables, cook until set.

Nutritional Value: ~200 calories per serving

Serving Suggestions:

1. Serve with a side of sliced tomatoes.
2. Enjoy with a cup of herbal tea.

Recipe 18: High-Calorie Shepherd's Pie

Ingredients:

- 500g ground lamb or beef
- 1 onion, diced
- 2 carrots, diced
- 1 cup peas

- 2 tbsp tomato paste
- 1 cup beef broth
- 3 cups mashed potatoes
- Salt and pepper to taste

Instructions:

1. Brown meat with onion and carrots.
2. Add peas, tomato paste, and broth, simmer until thickened.
3. Top with mashed potatoes, bake at 375°F for 20 minutes.

Nutritional Value: ~800 calories per serving

Serving Suggestions:

1. Pair with a side of steamed green beans.
2. Enjoy with a pint of stout beer.

Recipe 19: Low-Calorie Cauliflower Pizza

Ingredients:

- 1 cauliflower crust
- ¼ cup tomato sauce
- ½ cup shredded mozzarella cheese
- ½ bell pepper, sliced
- ¼ onion, sliced
- ¼ cup mushrooms, sliced

- Fresh basil for topping

Instructions:

1. Spread tomato sauce on cauliflower crust.

2. Top with cheese, bell pepper, onion, and mushrooms.

3. Bake according to crust instructions, garnish with basil.

Nutritional Value: ~400 calories per serving

Serving Suggestions:

1. Serve with a side of mixed greens with balsamic vinaigrette.

2. Pair with a glass of sparkling water with a slice of lemon.

Recipe 20: High-Calorie Creamy Seafood Pasta

Ingredients:

- 200g mixed seafood (shrimp, scallops, squid)

- 2 cups cooked linguine

- ½ cup heavy cream

- ¼ cup Parmesan cheese

- 2 garlic cloves, minced

- Salt and pepper to taste

- 1 tbsp olive oil

- Fresh parsley for garnish

-

Instructions:

1. Sauté seafood and garlic in olive oil.

2. Add cream and Parmesan cheese, simmer until thickened.

3. Toss in cooked pasta, season with salt and pepper.

4. Garnish with parsley.

Nutritional Value: ~750 calories per serving

Serving Suggestions:

1. Serve with a side of garlic bread.

2. Pair with a glass of white wine.

Recipe 21: Low-Calorie Stuffed Portobello Mushrooms

Ingredients:

- 4 large portobello mushrooms, stems removed

- 1 cup spinach, chopped

- ½ cup ricotta cheese

- 1/4 cup grated Parmesan

- 1 garlic clove, minced

- Salt and pepper to taste

- 1 tbsp olive oil

Instructions:

1. Mix spinach, ricotta, Parmesan, garlic, salt, and pepper.

2. Stuff mushrooms with the mixture.

3. Drizzle with olive oil and bake at 375°F for 20 minutes.

Nutritional Value: ~250 calories per serving

Serving Suggestions:

1. Pair with a side salad of mixed greens.

2. Enjoy with a glass of flavoured sparkling water.

Recipe 22: High-Calorie Pork Loin Roast with Vegetables

Ingredients: 500g pork loin roast

- 1 cup carrots, sliced

- 1 cup potatoes, cubed

- 1 onion, chopped

- 2 garlic cloves, minced

- 1 tbsp olive oil

- Salt, pepper, and rosemary to taste

Instructions:

1. Season pork with salt, pepper, and rosemary.

2. Roast with vegetables coated in olive oil at 375°F for 60 minutes.

Nutritional Value: ~700 calories per serving

Serving Suggestions:

1. Serve with a side of applesauce.

2. Pair with a glass of full-bodied red wine.

Recipe 23: Low-Calorie Garlic Shrimp Zoodles

Ingredients:

- 200g shrimp, peeled and deveined

- 2 zucchinis, spiralized

- 2 garlic cloves, minced

- 1 lemon, juice and zest

- Salt and pepper to taste

- 1 tbsp olive oil

- Fresh parsley for garnish

Instructions:

1. Sauté shrimp with garlic and lemon juice in olive oil.

2. Toss in zoodles, cook for 2-3 minutes.

3. Season with salt, pepper, and lemon zest.

4. Garnish with parsley.

Nutritional Value: ~300 calories per serving

Serving Suggestions:

1. Accompany with a side of steamed broccoli.

2. Enjoy with a glass of white wine.

Recipe 24: High-Calorie Chicken Parmesan

Ingredients: 2 chicken breasts, pounded thin

- 1 cup breadcrumbs

- ½ cup Parmesan cheese, grated

- 1 cup marinara sauce

- 1 cup mozzarella cheese, shredded

- Salt and pepper to taste

- 1 egg, beaten

- Olive oil for frying

Instructions:

1. Mix breadcrumbs with Parmesan, salt, and pepper.

2. Dip chicken in egg, then breadcrumb mixture.

3. Fry in olive oil until golden, transfer to baking dish.

4. Top with marinara and mozzarella, bake at 375°F for 20 minutes.

Nutritional Value: ~800 calories per serving

Serving Suggestions:

1. Serve with a side of spaghetti.

2. Pair with a Caesar salad.

Recipe 25: Low-Calorie Veggie Lentil Soup

Ingredients:

- 1 cup lentils
- 4 cups vegetable broth
- 1 carrot, diced
- 1 celery stalk, diced
- 1 onion, diced
- 2 garlic cloves, minced
- 1 tsp cumin
- Salt and pepper to taste
- 1 tbsp olive oil

Instructions:

1. Sauté onion, carrot, celery, and garlic in olive oil.
2. Add lentils, broth, and cumin, simmer until lentils are tender.
3. Season with salt and pepper.

Nutritional Value: ~350 calories per serving

Serving Suggestions:

1. Enjoy with a slice of whole-grain bread.
2. Pair with a side of mixed greens.

Recipe 26: High-Calorie Beef Lasagna Roll-Ups

Ingredients:

- 8 lasagna noodles, cooked
- 500g ground beef
- 1 cup ricotta cheese
- ½ cup Parmesan cheese
- 2 cups marinara sauce
- 1 egg
- Salt, pepper, and Italian seasoning

Instructions:

1. Brown beef, season with salt, pepper, and Italian seasoning.
2. Mix ricotta, Parmesan, and egg.
3. Spread ricotta mixture on noodles, top with beef, roll up.
4. Place in baking dish, cover with marinara sauce.
5. Bake at 375°F for 25 minutes.

Nutritional Value: ~800 calories per serving

Serving Suggestions:

1. Serve with a side of garlic bread.
2. Enjoy with a glass of red wine.

Recipe 27: Low-Calorie Grilled Fish Tacos

Ingredients:

- 2 white fish fillets
- 4 corn tortillas
- 1/2 cabbage, shredded
- ¼ cup Greek yogurt
- 1 lime, juiced
- 1 tbsp taco seasoning
- Salt and pepper to taste
- Fresh cilantro for garnish

Instructions:

1. Season fish with taco seasoning, grill until cooked.
2. Mix yogurt with lime juice, salt, and pepper.
3. Assemble tacos with fish, cabbage, and yogurt sauce.
4. Garnish with cilantro.

Nutritional Value: ~300 calories per serving

Serving Suggestions:

1. Pair with a side of black beans.
2. Enjoy with a glass of iced tea.

Recipe 28: High-Calorie Chicken and Bacon Carbonara

Ingredients: 2 cups cooked spaghetti

- 2 chicken breasts, cooked and sliced
- 4 bacon strips, cooked and chopped
- 2 eggs
- ½ cup Parmesan cheese
- 1 garlic clove, minced
- Salt and pepper to taste

Instructions:

1. Whisk eggs with Parmesan, garlic, salt, and pepper.
2. Toss spaghetti with egg mixture, chicken, and bacon.
3. Heat gently until sauce thickens.

Nutritional Value: ~700 calories per serving

Serving Suggestions:

1. Serve with a side of Caesar salad.
2. Pair with a glass of Chardonnay.

Recipe 29: Low-Calorie Baked Ratatouille

Ingredients:

- 1 zucchini, sliced
- 1 eggplant, sliced

- 2 tomatoes, sliced

- 1 bell pepper, sliced

- 1 onion, sliced

- 2 garlic cloves, minced

- ¼ cup tomato sauce

- Herbes de Provence, salt, and pepper

- 1 tbsp olive oil

Instructions:

1. Spread tomato sauce in baking dish.

2. Arrange vegetables in alternating patterns.

3. Drizzle with olive oil, season with herbs, garlic, salt, and pepper.

4. Bake at 375°F for 45 minutes.

Nutritional Value: ~200 calories per serving

Serving Suggestions:

1. Top with a sprinkle of grated Parmesan.

2. Enjoy with a glass of red wine.

Recipe 30: High-Calorie Sausage and Peppers

Ingredients:

- 4 Italian sausages

- 2 bell peppers, sliced

- 1 onion, sliced

- 2 garlic cloves, minced

- 1 cup marinara sauce

- Salt and pepper to taste

- 1 tbsp olive oil

Instructions:

1. Brown sausages in olive oil, remove and set aside.

2. Sauté peppers, onion, and garlic.

3. Add marinara sauce, return sausages to pan, simmer.

Nutritional Value: ~600 calories per serving

Serving Suggestions:

1. Serve over a bed of polenta.

2. Pair with a cold lager.

Recipe 31: Low-Calorie Cauliflower Fried Rice

Ingredients:

- 2 cups cauliflower rice

- 1 cup mixed vegetables (peas, carrots, corn)

- 2 eggs, beaten

- 2 tbsp soy sauce

- 1 garlic clove, minced

- 1 tsp sesame oil
- Green onions for garnish

Instructions:

1. Sauté vegetables and garlic in sesame oil.
2. Add cauliflower rice, cook for 5 minutes.
3. Push rice to the side, scramble eggs in the pan.
4. Mix everything together, add soy sauce.

Nutritional Value: ~250 calories per serving

Serving Suggestions:

1. Top with chopped green onions.
2. Enjoy with a cup of miso soup.

Recipe 32: High-Calorie Shrimp and Grits

Ingredients:

- 200g shrimp, peeled and deveined
- 1 cup grits, cooked
- ½ cup cheddar cheese
- 2 bacon strips, cooked and chopped
- ¼ cup green onions, chopped
- 1 garlic clove, minced
- Salt and pepper to taste
- 1 tbsp butter

Instructions:

1. Cook shrimp with garlic and butter.

2. Stir cheddar and bacon into cooked grits.

3. Serve shrimp over grits, garnish with green onions.

Nutritional Value: ~700 calories per serving

Serving Suggestions:

1. Serve with a side of sautéed spinach.

2. Pair with a glass of white wine

Dessert Recipes

Recipe 1: Low-Calorie Berry Yogurt Parfait

Ingredients:

- 1 cup Greek yogurt, low-fat
- ½ cup mixed berries (strawberries, blueberries)
- 1 tbsp honey
- A sprinkle of granola

Instructions:

1. Layer yogurt and berries in a glass.
2. Drizzle with honey and top with a sprinkle of granola.

Nutritional Value: ~200 calories per serving

Serving Suggestions:

1. Garnish with fresh mint leaves.
2. Pair with a cup of herbal tea for a light snack.

Recipe 2: High-Calorie Chocolate Lava Cake

Ingredients:

- 100g dark chocolate
- 100g butter
- 2 eggs
- ¼ cup sugar
- ¼ cup all-purpose flour

- 1 tsp vanilla extract

Instructions:

1. Melt chocolate and butter together.

2. Whisk eggs, sugar, and vanilla, then fold in chocolate mixture and flour.

3. Pour into greased ramekins and bake at 375°F for 12 minutes.

Nutritional Value: ~450 calories per serving

Serving Suggestions:

1. Serve with a scoop of vanilla ice cream.

2. Dust with powdered sugar.

Recipe 3: Low-Calorie Chia Seed Pudding

Ingredients:

- 3 tbsp chia seeds

- 1 cup almond milk, unsweetened

- 1 tsp vanilla extract

- 1 tbsp maple syrup

Instructions:

1. Mix chia seeds, almond milk, vanilla, and maple syrup.

2. Refrigerate overnight until set.

Nutritional Value: ~150 calories per serving

Serving Suggestions:

1. Top with a few slices of banana.

2. Enjoy with a small handful of nuts for added crunch.

Recipe 4: High-Calorie Tiramisu

Ingredients:

- 1 cup mascarpone cheese

- 1/2 cup heavy cream

- 1/4 cup sugar

- 1 cup espresso, cooled

- 12 ladyfingers

- Cocoa powder for dusting

Instructions:

1. Whip mascarpone, cream, and sugar until smooth.

2. Dip ladyfingers in espresso, layer in a dish.

3. Spread mascarpone mixture over ladyfingers, repeat layers.

4. Dust with cocoa powder and refrigerate for a few hours.

Nutritional Value: ~500 calories per serving

Serving Suggestions:

1. Garnish with chocolate shavings.

2. Pair with a small espresso to enhance the coffee flavour.

Recipe 5: Low-Calorie Fruit Sorbet

Ingredients:

- 2 cups frozen mixed fruit (mango, berries)

- 2 tbsp honey

- Juice of 1 lemon

Instructions:

1. Blend frozen fruit, honey, and lemon juice until smooth.

2. Freeze until set.

Nutritional Value: ~100 calories per serving

Serving Suggestions:

1. Garnish with fresh mint.

2. Serve as a refreshing palate cleanser after a meal.

Recipe 6: High-Calorie Pecan Pie

Ingredients:

- 1 pie crust

- 1 cup pecans, chopped

- 3 eggs

- 1 cup corn syrup

- ½ up brown sugar

- 2 tbsp butter, melted

- 1 tsp vanilla extract

Instructions:

1. Preheat oven to 350°F.

2. Mix eggs, corn syrup, sugar, butter, and vanilla.

3. Stir in pecans, pour into pie crust.

4. Bake for about 50 minutes.

Nutritional Value: ~500 calories per serving

Serving Suggestions:

1. Top with whipped cream.

2. Serve with a scoop of vanilla ice cream.

Recipe 7: Low-Calorie Baked Apples

Ingredients:

- 2 apples, cored

- 2 tbsp oats

- 1 tsp cinnamon

- 1 tbsp honey

- A pinch of nutmeg

Instructions:

1. Mix oats, cinnamon, honey, and nutmeg.

2. Stuff apples with the mixture.

3. Bake at 375°F for 25 minutes.

Nutritional Value: ~150 calories per serving

Serving Suggestions:

1. Drizzle with a bit more honey if desired.

2. Serve with a dollop of Greek yogurt.

Recipe 8: High-Calorie Cheesecake

Ingredients:

- 1 ½ cups crushed graham crackers
- ¼ cup melted butter
- 2 cups cream cheese
- 1 cup sugar
- 3 eggs
- 1 tsp vanilla extract

Instructions:

1. Mix graham crackers and butter, press into a pie pan.

2. Beat cream cheese and sugar, add eggs and vanilla.

3. Pour over crust, bake at 325°F for 50 minutes.

Nutritional Value: ~550 calories per serving

Serving Suggestions:

1. Top with fresh berries or fruit compote.

2. Drizzle with caramel or chocolate sauce.

Recipe 9: Low-Calorie Pumpkin Mousse

Ingredients:

- 1 cup pumpkin puree

- ½ cup Greek yogurt, low-fat

- 2 tbsp maple syrup

- 1 tsp pumpkin pie spice

Instructions:

1. Mix pumpkin puree, yogurt, maple syrup, and pumpkin pie spice until smooth.

2. Refrigerate for an hour before serving.

Nutritional Value: ~120 calories per serving

Serving Suggestions:

1. Top with a sprinkle of cinnamon.

2. Serve with a few ginger snaps on the side.

Recipe 10: High-Calorie Banana Foster

Ingredients:

- 2 bananas, sliced

- 1/4 cup brown sugar

- 2 tbsp butter

- ¼ cup rum

- ½ tsp cinnamon

- Vanilla ice cream for serving

Instructions:

1. Melt butter in a pan, add sugar and cinnamon, cook until bubbly.

2. Add bananas and rum, cook until bananas are soft.

3. Serve hot over vanilla ice cream.

Nutritional Value: ~400 calories per serving

Serving Suggestions:

1. Sprinkle with chopped nuts for added texture.

2. Pair with a small cup of coffee or espresso.

Recipe 11: Low-Calorie Peach Cobbler

Ingredients: 2 peaches, sliced

- ¼ cup almond flour

- 1 tbsp coconut oil

- 1 tbsp honey

- 1/2 tsp cinnamon

- A pinch of nutmeg

Instructions:

1. Arrange peach slices in a baking dish.

2. Mix almond flour, coconut oil, honey, cinnamon, and nutmeg; sprinkle over peaches.

3. Bake at 375°F for 20 minutes.

Nutritional Value: ~200 calories per serving

Serving Suggestions:

1. Top with a dollop of Greek yogurt.

2. Serve with a cup of chamomile tea for a comforting dessert.

Recipe 12: High-Calorie Chocolate Mousse

Ingredients:

- 100g dark chocolate

- 2 eggs, separated

- ¼ cup sugar

- ½ cup heavy cream

- 1 tsp vanilla extract

Instructions:

1. Melt chocolate and let it cool slightly.

2. Whip egg whites until stiff peaks form.

3. Beat egg yolks with sugar, then mix into chocolate.

4. Fold in egg whites and whipped cream.

5. Refrigerate for at least 2 hours.

Nutritional Value: ~400 calories per serving

Serving Suggestions:

1. Garnish with fresh raspberries or strawberries.

2. Pair with a small glass of dessert wine.

Recipe 13: Low-Calorie Carrot Cake Cupcakes

Ingredients: 1 cup grated carrots

- ½ cup almond flour

- ¼ cup applesauce

- 2 eggs

- ¼ cup honey

- 1 tsp cinnamon

- ½ tsp baking soda

Instructions:

1. Mix all ingredients until well combined.

2. Pour into lined cupcake tins.

3. Bake at 350°F for 20-25 minutes.

Nutritional Value: ~150 calories per serving

Serving Suggestions:

1. Top with a thin layer of low-fat cream cheese frosting.

2. Serve with a cup of ginger tea for a spicy complement.

Recipe 14: High-Calorie Apple Pie

Ingredients: Pie crust

- 4 apples, peeled and sliced
- ½ cup sugar
- 2 tbsp butter
- 1 tsp cinnamon
- ¼ tsp nutmeg
- 1 tbsp flour

Instructions:

1. Toss apples with sugar, cinnamon, nutmeg, and flour.
2. Fill pie crust with apple mixture, dot with butter.
3. Cover with top crust, bake at 375°F for 50 minutes.

Nutritional Value: ~500 calories per serving

Serving Suggestions:

1. Serve warm with a scoop of vanilla ice cream.
2. Enjoy with a cup of hot mulled cider.

Recipe 15: Low-Calorie Frozen Yogurt Bark

Ingredients:

- 2 cups Greek yogurt, low-fat
- 1 tbsp honey

- ½ cup mixed berries

- 2 tbsp dark chocolate chips

Instructions:

1. Spread yogurt on a baking sheet lined with parchment paper.

2. Drizzle with honey, sprinkle with berries and chocolate chips.

3. Freeze until solid, break into pieces.

Nutritional Value: ~100 calories per serving

Serving Suggestions:

1. Enjoy as a cool, refreshing snack on a hot day.

2. Serve as a light dessert at a summer gathering.

Recipe 16: High-Calorie Cheesecake Brownies

Ingredients:

- Brownie mix

- 1 cup cream cheese

- ¼ cup sugar

- 1 egg

- 1 tsp vanilla extract

Instructions:

1. Prepare brownie mix as per instructions.

2. Beat cream cheese with sugar, egg, and vanilla.

3. Pour brownie batter into a pan, top with cream cheese mixture.

4. Swirl with a knife, bake as per brownie instructions.

Nutritional Value: ~450 calories per serving

Serving Suggestions:

1. Top with a dollop of whipped cream.

2. Serve with a glass of cold milk.

Recipe 17: Low-Calorie Banana Ice Cream

Ingredients:

- 2 frozen bananas
- ¼ cup almond milk
- 1 tsp vanilla extract
- A pinch of cinnamon

Instructions:

1. Blend frozen bananas with almond milk and vanilla until smooth.

2. Freeze until it reaches desired consistency.

Nutritional Value: ~120 calories per serving

Serving Suggestions:

1. Top with a sprinkle of granola for crunch.

2. Pair with a few dark chocolate shavings for extra indulgence.

Recipe 18: High-Calorie Pecan Sticky Buns

Ingredients:

- 1 can refrigerated biscuit dough
- ½ cup brown sugar
- ¼ cup butter
- ½ cup chopped pecans
- 1 tsp cinnamon

Instructions:

1. Melt butter with brown sugar and cinnamon, pour into baking dish.
2. Place biscuits on top, sprinkle with pecans.
3. Bake as per biscuit instructions.

Nutritional Value: ~500 calories per serving

Serving Suggestions:

1. Serve warm, fresh out of the oven.
2. Enjoy with a cup of strong coffee.

Recipe 19: Low-Calorie Mixed Berry Compote

Ingredients:

- 2 cups mixed berries (fresh or frozen)
- 2 tbsp honey

- 1 tsp lemon juice

Instructions:

1. Simmer berries, honey, and lemon juice until thickened.

2. Let cool before serving.

Nutritional Value: ~100 calories per serving

Serving Suggestions:

1. Serve over low-fat Greek yogurt.

2. Use as a topping for whole-grain pancakes or waffles.

Recipe 20: High-Calorie Molten Chocolate Cakes

Ingredients:

- 100g dark chocolate

- 100g butter

- 2 eggs

- 2 egg yolks

- 1/4 cup sugar

- 2 tbsp flour

- 1 tsp vanilla extract

Instructions:

1. Melt chocolate and butter together.

2. Whisk eggs, egg yolks, sugar, and vanilla, then fold in chocolate mixture and flour.

3. Pour into greased ramekins and bake at 375°F for 12 minutes.

Nutritional Value: ~450 calories per serving

Serving Suggestions:

1. Serve with a scoop of raspberry sorbet.

2. Accompany with a small glass of port wine.

Recipe 21: Low-Calorie Avocado Chocolate Mousse

Ingredients:

- 1 ripe avocado

- 2 tbsp unsweetened cocoa powder

- 2 tbsp honey or maple syrup

- ½ tsp vanilla extract

- A pinch of salt

- Almond milk (as needed for consistency)

Instructions:

1. Blend avocado, cocoa powder, honey/maple syrup, vanilla, and salt until smooth.

2. Add almond milk as needed for desired consistency.

3. Chill before serving.

Nutritional Value: ~200 calories per serving

Serving Suggestions:

1. Garnish with a few raspberries.

2. Serve as a dip with fresh fruit slices.

Recipe 22: High-Calorie Raspberry Cheesecake

Ingredients:

- 1 ½ cups crushed graham crackers

- ¼ cup melted butter

- 2 cups cream cheese

- 1 cup sugar

- 3 eggs

- 1 tsp vanilla extract

- 1 cup raspberries

Instructions:

1. Mix graham crackers and butter, press into a pie pan.

2. Beat cream cheese and sugar, add eggs and vanilla.

3. Pour over crust, top with raspberries.

4. Bake at 325°F for 50 minutes.

Nutritional Value: ~550 calories per serving

Serving Suggestions:

1. Top with whipped cream.

2. Serve with a small scoop of raspberry sorbet.

Recipe 23: Low-Calorie Watermelon Granita

Ingredients:

- 4 cups cubed watermelon
- Juice of 1 lime
- 1 tbsp honey

Instructions:

1. Blend watermelon, lime juice, and honey.
2. Freeze mixture, scraping with a fork every hour until slushy.

Nutritional Value: ~100 calories per serving

Serving Suggestions:

1. Garnish with a sprig of mint.
2. Serve as a refreshing end to a summer meal.

Recipe 24: High-Calorie Banana Nut Bread

Ingredients:

- 3 ripe bananas, mashed
- 1/3 cup melted butter
- ½ cup sugar
- 1 egg, beaten
- 1 tsp vanilla extract

- 1 tsp baking soda

- 1 ½ cups all-purpose flour

- ½ cup walnuts, chopped

Instructions:

1. Mix bananas with butter, sugar, egg, and vanilla.

2. Add baking soda and flour, fold in walnuts.

3. Pour into a greased loaf pan, bake at 350°F for 50-60 minutes.

Nutritional Value: ~350 calories per slice

Serving Suggestions:

1. Serve warm with a pat of butter.

2. Enjoy with a cup of hot tea or coffee.

Recipe 25: Low-Calorie Strawberry Sorbet

Ingredients:

- 2 cups frozen strawberries

- 2 tbsp honey

- Juice of 1 lemon

Instructions:

1. Blend strawberries, honey, and lemon juice until smooth.

2. Freeze until set, stirring occasionally.

Nutritional Value: ~120 calories per serving

Serving Suggestions:

1. Garnish with fresh mint leaves.

2. Serve between courses as a palate cleanser.

Recipe 26: High-Calorie Profiteroles

Ingredients:

- 1 cup water

- ½ cup butter

- 1 cup all-purpose flour

- 4 eggs

- 1 cup heavy cream, whipped

- Chocolate sauce

Instructions:

1. Boil water and butter, stir in flour. Cook until mixture forms a ball.

2. Remove from heat, beat in eggs one at a time.

3. Drop by spoonful onto a baking sheet, bake at 425°F for 20-25 minutes.

4. Fill with whipped cream, drizzle with chocolate sauce.

Nutritional Value: ~400 calories per serving

Serving Suggestions:

1. Dust with powdered sugar.

2. Serve with a small cup of espresso.

Recipe 27: Low-Calorie Pineapple Coconut Bars

Ingredients:

- 2 cups chopped pineapple
- 1 cup unsweetened shredded coconut
- ¼ cup almond flour
- 2 eggs
- 1 tbsp honey

Instructions:

1. Mix all ingredients and press into a lined baking dish.
2. Bake at 350°F for 30 minutes.
3. Cool and slice into bars.

Nutritional Value: ~150 calories per serving

Serving Suggestions:

1. Enjoy as a tropical snack.
2. Pair with a cup of green tea.

Recipe 28: High-Calorie Chocolate Chip Cookies

Ingredients:

- ½ cup butter, softened
- ½ cup sugar
- ½ cup brown sugar

- 1 egg

- 1 tsp vanilla extract

- 1 ½ cups all-purpose flour

- ½ tsp baking soda

- 1 cup chocolate chips

Instructions:

1. Cream butter and sugars, beat in egg and vanilla.

2. Mix in flour and baking soda, stir in chocolate chips.

3. Drop spoonful on a baking sheet, bake at 375°F for 10 minutes.

Nutritional Value: ~300 calories per cookie

Serving Suggestions:

1. Serve with a glass of cold milk.

2. Enjoy as a comforting treat with hot cocoa.

Recipe 29: Low-Calorie Mixed Berry Compote with Greek Yogurt

Ingredients:

- 2 cups mixed berries (fresh or frozen)

- 2 tbsp honey

- 1 cup Greek yogurt, low-fat

Instructions:

1. Simmer berries and honey until thickened.

2. Let cool and serve over Greek yogurt.

Nutritional Value: ~200 calories per serving

Serving Suggestions:

1. Top with a sprinkle of granola.

2. Serve as a healthy breakfast alternative.

Recipe 30: High-Calorie Salted Caramel Brownies

Ingredients:

- ½ cup butter
- 1 cup sugar
- 2 eggs
- 1 tsp vanilla extract
- 1/3 cup unsweetened cocoa powder
- ½ cup all-purpose flour
- ¼ tsp salt
- ¼ tsp baking powder
- Salted caramel sauce for topping

Instructions:

1. Mix butter, sugar, eggs, and vanilla.

2. Stir in cocoa, flour, salt, and baking powder.

3. Pour into a greased pan, bake at 350°F for 25-30 minutes.

4. Drizzle with salted caramel sauce.

Nutritional Value: ~350 calories per serving

Serving Suggestions:

1. Serve warm with a scoop of vanilla ice cream.

2. Pair with a cup of freshly brewed coffee.

Recipe 31: Low-Calorie Frozen Banana Bites

Ingredients:

- 2 bananas, sliced

- ¼ cup dark chocolate, melted

- ¼ cup peanut butter, melted

Instructions:

1. Sandwich banana slices with peanut butter, freeze until firm.

2. Dip in melted chocolate, freeze again until set.

Nutritional Value: ~100 calories per serving

Serving Suggestions:

1. Enjoy as a quick, healthy snack.

2. Serve at a kids' party for a healthier treat option.

Recipe 32: High-Calorie Lemon Pound Cake

Ingredients:

- 1 cup butter, softened
- 1 cup sugar
- 4 eggs
- 1 tsp vanilla extract
- 2 cups all-purpose flour
- 1 lemon, zest and juice
- ¼ cup milk

Instructions:

1. Cream butter and sugar, add eggs and vanilla.
2. Mix in flour, lemon zest, juice, and milk.
3. Bake in a loaf pan at 350°F for 60 minutes.

Nutritional Value: ~450 calories per serving

Serving Suggestions:

1. Glaze with a lemon icing.
2. Serve with a dollop of whipped cream.

Recipe 33: Low-Calorie Apple Cinnamon Chips

Ingredients:

- 2 apples, thinly sliced
- 1 tsp cinnamon

- 1 tbsp sugar

Instructions:

1. Toss apple slices with cinnamon and sugar.

2. Arrange on a baking sheet, bake at 200°F for 2 hours.

Nutritional Value: ~50 calories per serving

Serving Suggestions:

1. Crunchy snack on its own.

2. Sprinkle over oatmeal or yogurt.

These dessert recipes offer a balance of indulgent and lighter options, perfect for different days in a Metabolic Confusion diet. They cater to various tastes while keeping nutritional considerations in mind.

Sample Meal Plan

Week 1 Meal Plan

Day 1 (High-Calorie)

- **Breakfast**: High-Calorie Avocado Toast

- **Lunch**: High-Calorie Beef Stir-Fry

- **Dinner**: High-Calorie Pork Chop with Apple Sauce

- **Dessert**: High-Calorie Chocolate Lava Cake

Day 2 (Low-Calorie)

- **Breakfast**: Low-Calorie Berry Smoothie

- **Lunch**: Low-Calorie Cauliflower Rice Bowl

- **Dinner**: Low-Calorie Grilled Salmon with Asparagus

- **Dessert**: Low-Calorie Peach Cobbler

Day 3 (High-Calorie)

- **Breakfast**: High-Calorie Protein-Packed Breakfast Bowl

- **Lunch**: High-Calorie Chicken Caesar Wrap

- **Dinner**: High-Calorie Chicken Alfredo Pasta

- **Dessert**: High-Calorie Tiramisu

Day 4 (Low-Calorie)

- **Breakfast**: Low-Calorie Greek Yogurt Parfait

- **Lunch**: Low-Calorie Turkey Lettuce Wraps

- **Dinner**: Low-Calorie Baked Cod with Lemon and Herbs

- **Dessert**: Low-Calorie Chia Seed Pudding

Day 5 (High-Calorie)

- **Breakfast**: High-Calorie Breakfast Burrito

- **Lunch**: High-Calorie Tuna Pasta Salad

- **Dinner**: High-Calorie Shepherd's Pie

- **Dessert**: High-Calorie Pecan Pie

Day 6 (Low-Calorie)

- **Breakfast**: Low-Calorie Oatmeal

- **Lunch**: Low-Calorie Mediterranean Chickpea Salad

- **Dinner**: Low-Calorie Vegetable Curry

- **Dessert**: Low-Calorie Watermelon Granita

Day 7 (High-Calorie)

- **Breakfast**: High-Calorie Breakfast Tacos

- **Lunch**: High-Calorie Sausage and Peppers

- **Dinner**: High-Calorie Beef Chili

- **Dessert**: High-Calorie Cheesecake Brownies

General Guidelines:

- **High-Calorie Days**: Focus on more energy-dense foods, including healthy fats and proteins.

- **Low-Calorie Days**: Emphasize vegetables, lean proteins, and lower-calorie fruits.

- **Desserts**: Chosen to complement the calorie goals of each day while providing a satisfying end to the meal.

CONCLUSION

At its core, Metabolic Confusion is based on the premise that alternating between higher and lower calorie days can prevent the body from adapting to a consistent caloric intake, thereby potentially enhancing metabolism and aiding in weight loss or management. This approach contrasts with traditional dieting methods, which often involve a consistent caloric deficit or specific macronutrient distribution. The primary aim is to circumvent the plateau effect commonly seen in traditional diets, where the body adapts to reduced calorie intake, and weight loss slows down or stops. By varying calorie intake, the body may not adapt as easily, potentially avoiding or reducing the plateau effect in weight loss. Additionally, this method is proposed to impact the hormonal responses related to hunger and satiety, such as ghrelin and leptin, potentially aiding in appetite control on low-calorie days.

However, it's crucial to address the myths surrounding Metabolic Confusion. It does not guarantee rapid or effortless weight loss, nor does it dramatically boost metabolism leading to higher calorie burning at rest. The effectiveness of the diet is not uniform across all individuals, and the quality of the diet in terms of nutrient density and variety remains paramount for overall health. The diet's flexibility and psychological ease are among its most significant benefits, offering a break from the stricter low-calorie periods, which can make the diet easier to adhere to for some people.

In terms of recipe creation, the focus was on developing a wide range of meal options that cater to both high and low-calorie days as part of the Metabolic Confusion Diet. The breakfast recipes ranged from nutrient-dense smoothies and yogurt parfaits to more indulgent options like avocado toast and protein-packed breakfast bowls. Lunch recipes included lighter choices like salads and soups, as well as heartier meals like pasta and stir-fries. Dinner recipes were a mix of low-calorie options like grilled fish and vegetable stir-fry, and higher-calorie comfort foods like lasagna and chili. The dessert recipes were designed to complement the calorie goals of each day, from light and refreshing fruit-based treats to richer, more decadent options like chocolate mousse and cheesecake.

The 7-day sample meal plan was a culmination of this recipe creation process, demonstrating how the meals could be combined and rotated to adhere to the principles of Metabolic Confusion. The plan aimed to offer a balanced and diverse array of meals, ensuring a mix of different protein sources, vegetables, and flavours. It also emphasized the importance of adjusting portion sizes and ingredients to align with individual calorie needs and dietary goals.

Throughout the discussion, it was evident that while Metabolic Confusion offers a novel approach to dieting, it requires careful planning and consideration. The diet's flexibility, which is one of its main appeals, can also be a challenge, as it demands a good understanding of nutritional content and portion sizes. Furthermore, it's essential to note that individual experiences and results may vary widely. What works for one person might not be as effective for another, and personal preferences, lifestyle, and specific health conditions must be taken into account. As with any dietary approach, consulting healthcare professionals, particularly for those with specific health conditions or nutritional concerns, is crucial.

In conclusion, the Metabolic Confusion Diet presents an intriguing alternative to traditional constant-calorie diets. By incorporating fluctuating caloric intake, it aims to prevent metabolic adaptation, potentially avoiding weight loss plateaus and providing a more sustainable and psychologically satisfying approach to weight management. However, the effectiveness and suitability of this diet can vary widely among individuals. It's important to maintain a balanced, nutrient-rich diet and to consult healthcare professionals for personalized dietary advice. Future research is needed to fully understand and validate the effects and mechanisms of Metabolic Confusion in weight management. As with any diet, the key is finding a balanced approach that aligns with individual health needs, preferences, and lifestyles, and adapting and fine-tuning the approach over time for sustainability and effectiveness.